Tough Times!

Tough Times!

Dalia Burton

iUniverse, Inc.
New York Bloomington Shanghai

Tough Times!

iUniverse books may be ordered through booksellers or by contacting:

iUniverse
1663 Liberty Drive
Bloomington, IN 47403
www.iuniverse.com
1-800-Authors (1-800-288-4677)

ISBN: 978-0-595-49680-8 (pbk)
ISBN: 978-0-595-61207-9 (ebk)

Printed in the United States of America

Contents

THANKS TO

REBECCA NICOLE BURTON, My Daughter, hoping you will never have to endure what I have endured and if someday you should have to go through this experience, I leave you this book to guide and help you, to give you the strength that I had to draw upon. I am proud of you, always encouraging me, you are the light of my life, my all. I love you with all my heart. God bless you sweetheart.

TRACE BURTON, My Husband, thanks for all the support you gave me during my battle with breast cancer.

IGNACIA DE LAIN, My Mother, for being with me day and night. For sharing my anguish and sadness, for always lifting my spirits, for cooking my favorite Venezuelan dishes and helping me maintain my weight. Forgive me for causing you so many tears and sadness. I know you suffered as much as I did. I give thanks to God for letting us be together. Mama, one and a million thanks, I could not have made it without you. You shared my tears, my fears, and my pain. Thank you for being at the core of my happiness, I love you from the bottom of my heart.

REVECA COOPER, My Sister, for sharing with me the moments I considered the most difficult, the beginning of this battle. Thank you for always being there for me, you provided much of my strength, for unconditional love, for simply being my best friend.

SAM, NORMA AND THEIR DAUGHTER SHERRI, My in-Laws, for always being there unconditionally, for taking care of my Daughter and Me, for being with me during some of my treatments, for always looking out for me.

GARY COOPER, My Brother-in-Law, for what we have in common, for always having answers to all of my questions and for calming my anxieties, always making me laugh and teaching me patience.

CESAR, SORAYA, IRMA, My Brother and Sisters, even though we were far from each other, I felt you near, for your concerns, for keeping me in your prayers and for helping me stay positive.

ALICIA, My Cousin, for helping me stay beautiful, for helping me even out my lack of hair. You are a very special cousin and friend and I wish you all the best in the world because you deserve it. For always being there for me when I needed you and even when I didn't (ha-ha).

ESTER, My Cousin, I want to tell you that I have my refrigerator full of sodas (ha-ha). Thank you for all the advice you've given me. I am happy we are in contact with each other again, you are not going to get away from me even if you try.

To My Ant Teresa and My Godmother Lala, Thank you so much for all the support that I got from you, for always calling and keeping me and my Moms' spirit up, thank you so much.

MY FRIENDS, Michele Lamb, Christine Marshall, Jen Steel, Lanie Koziel, Janie Graham, Diane Schiesl, Gloria Howard. Thank you all for keeping me in your prayers. Special thanks to one of my best friends: Trish Magnusson and her beautiful family, your support meant so much to me. To Virginia, for making my dream come true, thank you so much for your time. To Mymiri, the main reason why I always wanted to look beautiful, you will always be in my heart.

KLASSEN FAMILY, Dennis, Terri and Esther, for the unconditional help I received from all of you, words cannot express the gratitude I feel. I love you all and thank you for making me a part of your beautiful family, God bless you.

TO MY DOCTORS AND THEIR STAFF, Dr. Edward Hayashi, Dr. Deborah Villa, Dr. Jonathan Stella, for your care, time and patience, for keeping my spirits up, I am very happy to be in your hands.

CESAR LAIN BORDERAS, My Father, wherever you are, you gave me a boost, I have always felt you close by me, thank you from my heart for being with me day and night to protect me, to give me the wisdom to face this trial with strength and above all, patience.

This book is also dedicated to **ALL OF THE GOOD PEOPLE** who one day will hear those terrible words "You have cancer" and with the hope that this narrative may help you be yet one more survivor.

And finally, to the **ALL POWERFUL** for giving me a second chance in this life, I won't fail you.

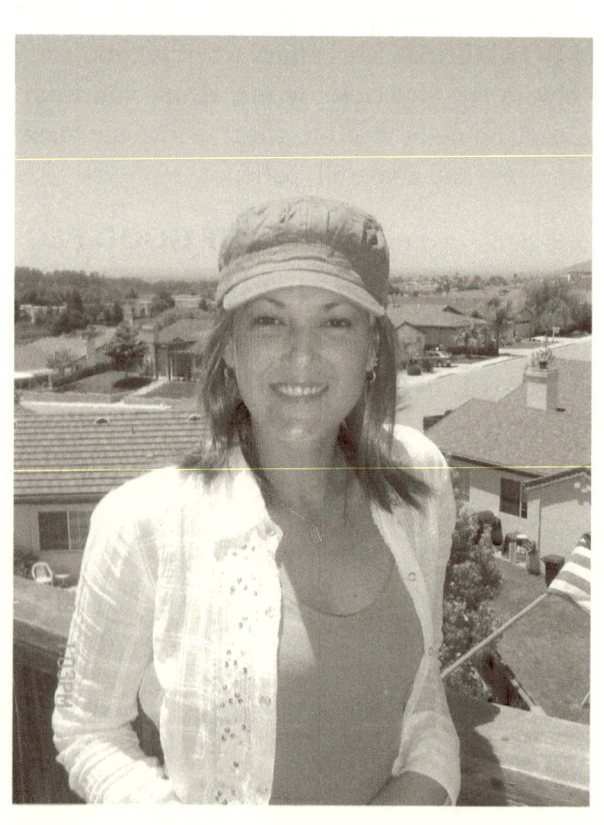

INTRODUCTION

When we speak of women, we refer to their beauty, be it physical or spiritual. It's so unbelievable to be able to see how grand woman is in the true sense of the world. We look at women in different parts of the world and we can realize they have different necessities in their lives. We realize also that women have many differing roles as a Woman, as a Wife, as a Daughter and above all, as a Mother. We can also see that in all stages in a woman's life come problems, anxieties, joys, burdens and some illnesses. We are going to explore these issues and focus more precisely on Breast Cancer. This illness does not discriminate due to race, creed, religion, economic level, or strength.

In this book, we'll speak of all the aspects of breast cancer and of vivid experiences. I am a woman who has survived this trial which I thought never could have happened. This is a real-life story. This illness came to me when there was so much happiness and tranquility in my life. It was then that I started on this path filled with anguish. We can appreciate that at the end of that path lies hope, that at the end of a long travel with the heavy burden of Breast Cancer one can still go forward and above all, one can deal with such a grave illness.

In this book, you will find the strength to walk that path of anguish, pain and above all the necessary strength to have hope. You will appreciate the emotional and physical changes during the operations and treatments as well as learn to bear them with much energy and bravery. And lastly, you will see you can conquer much sadness thanks to that bravery, your faith and the spirit to fight day-after-day. You will see emotional changes as well as physical ones, experiences and new attitudes that prove you will understand and enjoy life again. You will learn to endure, understand and most of all go forward with complete serenity during an illness that is a reality: Breast Cancer.

As with almost all forms of cancer, early detection will help receive effective treatment. One of the best methods is monthly self-examination. This method will allow you to learn the texture, conformity of the breast and notice any changes manifested. The most serious problem with breast cancer is that it can metasticize to other parts of the body. There are different types of breast cancer, some very aggressive, some less. They are also classified on different stages. Breast cancer treatment usually begins within a few weeks of diagnosis. During this time, you should consult with a surgeon and learn all you can related to surgical options and decide what is best for you. After having analyzed the type of treatment that's best, make your choice. The majority of women prefer to make their own decisions. After all, the type of surgery that you choose will affect the way you feel. Usually it's difficult to make a decision quickly and you may opt for a second opinion. This will enable you to make a clearer decision and give you the opportunity to discuss your case with another physician who may offer other options or reassure you that you have made the right choice. Getting a second opinion is better than worrying that you made a wrong or hasty decision.

When I learned that I had Breast Cancer, I experienced much anguish and had many questions. I had a lot to think about and I encountered many well-intentioned people to whom I am heartily grateful for teaching me to make my own decisions. People suggested that now was the time to change my diet, exercise more, and think of my Daughter, my home, and my life, aside from that, think about my surgeries, biopsies, results, chemotherapy, radiation, Doctors and so forth. I could not take it all at once, it was too much. I sat down logically and saw myself as a life-saving project: step-by-step. I realized that a library does not document facts without organizing alphabetically. That is exactly the way I made my decision, I took everything one-by-one and day-by-day.

I will tell you my experiences, how cancer changed my life physically and emotionally. I sustained many scars on my body. Many chemicals weakened me almost completely. I was fatigued to the point of completely impeding my daily life. But I can tell you that my soul was strengthened more every day. I will never ask The Almighty why. On the contrary, I will thank him for letting me see life the way I do now, and I am sure He'll do the same for you.

GOD NEVER SENDS YOU MORE THAN YOU CAN BEAR

1

DIAGNOSIS

It all started one morning while I was in the shower. During my routine breast check, I felt a lump in my left breast. I was immediately nervous and what came to mind was the illness that took my Father, cancer.

Thank God, for that reason, I took immediate action and called my Doctor for an appointment which was scheduled two weeks later. When I arrived, my Doctor did not seem too worried. First of all, I was only 36 years old and second the lump seemed small and well-defined, and third my medical history. The Doctor ordered a mammogram, something I thought I would not need for a few years. The Doctors' conclusion was a lump that would need further checking in 6 months.

Naturally, those results calmed me. I went on with my life as usual and even made a trip to Florida to visit my cousin Alicia. I enjoyed my visit and forgot everything. During the trip, I noticed that the lump started to grow rapidly.

Three months had passed since my first consultation, so I made another appointment with the Doctor and I clearly remember that the Doctor said that "it was nothing, the lump had definition". I said to my Doctor "I didn't care how well-defined my lump was, I wanted to get rid of it, I didn't like the way the lump was growing, and I was getting very nervous. So my Doctor ordered for my lump to be removed to relieve my worries. I had another mammogram, but this time it showed something different. The Doctors could not define the problem so they sug-

gested a biopsy. Inside I knew from those results that something was not right.

I was referred to a General Practicioner who told me he'd rather remove the lump to be analyzed in the laboratory rather than take only a small portion of the lump. I was in agreement.

The day of the surgery, I was very nervous but glad that I was finally going to be rid of the lump so that my breast would no longer be disfigured.

The operation took an hour-and-a-half. He removed the lump and a tumor that was growing alongside. He said that everything was all right. My recuperation went perfectly and in less than 2 days I was living a normal life, but I was really getting ready for what was only the start of a long journey.

I thank God today that I did not delay because if I had disregarded my instincts and done nothing it might have been too late. It's not true that if the tumor is well-defined it means that it is benign.

2

DEFINITION OF BREAST CANCER

Cancer is a group of cells that grow together in an uncontrollable manner invading and harming healthy tissue. A group of cancerous cells form a protuberance called a tumor. If a tumor is situated in the breast it is called breast cancer.

All of our organs and tissues consist of different types of cells. Our bodies stay healthy normally by the way the cells grow and renew and almost all cells need to be replaced at regular intervals. Normal and healthy cells grow, divide and die under gene control. If there is a change in the genes that control growth, a healthy cell will change into a malignant cell (tumor). These changes indicate that the cell will appear abnormal under a microscope. They change in shape and the cells appear different. They grow uncontrollably and divide into more and more cancerous cells. These tumors can be cancerous or benign. Benign tumors grow very slowly and do not spread to other parts of the body. Malignant tumors are dangerous and they grow faster and can spread to other parts of the body thus forming secondary tumors (metastasis).

2.1 TYPES-STAGES OF BREAST CANCER.

Doctors speak of stages of cancer. This is how they define the size of the tumors and how it has spread. If you are not aware of the type or stage of your cancer, ask your doctor or nurse.

TYPE 0: Means you have a CDIS or CLIS.

-CDIS (Carcinoma Ductal in Situ) occur when breast cancer is in the first stage and generally is so small that it does not form a mass. Your doctor may describe CDIS as non-invasive cancer

-CLIS (Lobal Carcinoma in Situ) is not cancer but may increase the risk of getting breast cancer.

STAGE 1: If your cancer measures less than 1 inch wide (2 centimeters) your cancer is found only in the breast and has not spread to the lymph nodes, part of the immune system in the body that helps combat infections and illnesses, or other parts of the body. This is the type that I have.

STAGE IIA:

-Breast cancer was not found, but was located in the glands found under the arms or

-the cancer measures 1 inch or less and has spread to the lymphatic nodes or

-your cancer measures approximately 1 or 2 inches (2 to 5 centimeters) but has not spread to the lymphatic nodes.

STAGE IIIA:

Cancer was not found in the breast, but was found in the lymphatic nodes present under the arm. They are connected to each other or

-The Cancer measures 2 inches (5 centimeters) or less and has spread to the under arm lymph nodes.

STAGE IIIB:

Means that the tumor may have grown inside the wall of the thorax, breast or lymph nodes.

-Inflammatory cancer of the breast is a type IIIB, it is rare, the breast appears red or swollen.

STAGE IIIC:

Means that the cancer has spread to the lymphatic nodes, in the armpit, or the glands above or below the clavicle. The primary tumor may be of any size.

STAGE IV:

Is further metastasis. The cancer has spread to other parts of the body. Recurring cancer is returned cancer after having been treated.

3

CONVERSATION WITH MY DAUGHTER

My daughter observed continuously my every movement, my telephone calls to the doctors and my making appointments. My face showed anguish and pain. She would look at me often but never asked questions. I realized she had the right to know. One fine day I sat down with her and delicately, using simple terms, not medical terms, told her that the doctor found a little ball in mommy's breast and the doctor had taken it out and that I will have to take much medicine to get well.

I told her that probably with all the medications that I was about to take, my hair would fall out and that I might feel somewhat ill. I also explained to her that this has nothing to do with her, no one was at fault, this was just something that happens, but I was going to fight to get well.

My daughter looked up at me and said "it doesn't matter what happens or that your hair will fall out, I love you so much for your outside but most of it for your inside." To this day I remember those words and I know I'll never forget them.

Then she told me that I was lucky because I'd never have to comb my hair and that we will save a lot of money on shampoo so in some way she envied me. I started to laugh and told her to cut her hair with me, she laughed back and said "no Mommy, my friends in school would make fun of me," so I said, "ahh so you're saying they will make fun of

6

me?" She laughed and replied "Mommy, but how are they going to make fun of you if you're too old to go to school?"

There were many days when I found myself in bed without the desire to do anything, where I felt very lonely and sorry for myself, nothing motivated me, I wanted to give up to the physical and mental pain. Whenever my daughter saw me like this, she would try to cheer me up and when that didn't work she would bring all her toys to my bed and declare "o.k. then we'll play here all day". She would prepare sandwiches that only she thought were delicious. It seems incredible how quickly children adapt to any situation. She called me her favorite baldy and when she saw me a little sad she would go to great lengths to make me laugh.

Daughter, you are the light of my life. Perhaps you are too young to understand now but all I want to say to you is that without you, my life would be very sad and empty. There is nothing I would change about you. You are perfect in my world. You will always be my baby. I am proud of you, you are the main reason for my fighting, you know why? Because I love you with all my heart.

IT IS VERY IMPORTANT TO:

-Plan what you're going to say and how you're going to say it.

-Avoid medical terms with them. Use only language your children can easily understand.

-Listen to your children to know what they've heard.

-Don't lie to them. Children know when you're hiding something.

-Correct erroneous thoughts that in their young minds they have created.

-Try and keep routines as normal as possible.

-Keep your child's school informed of your condition so they may be aware of any changes in his or her behavior.

-Be honest with your children, let them know how you feel.

-Remember it's perfectly normal to cry for yourself and your children.

-Prepare to repeat any questions or answer more than once.

-Don't be afraid to say "I don't know."

-Hide your emotions, it's the best thing to do.

-Don't use elaborate or medical terms.

-Don't make promises you can't keep.

Your children have the right to know things that can affect the family, for example a diagnosis of cancer. Try to always tell them the truth so they'll not seek answers elsewhere.

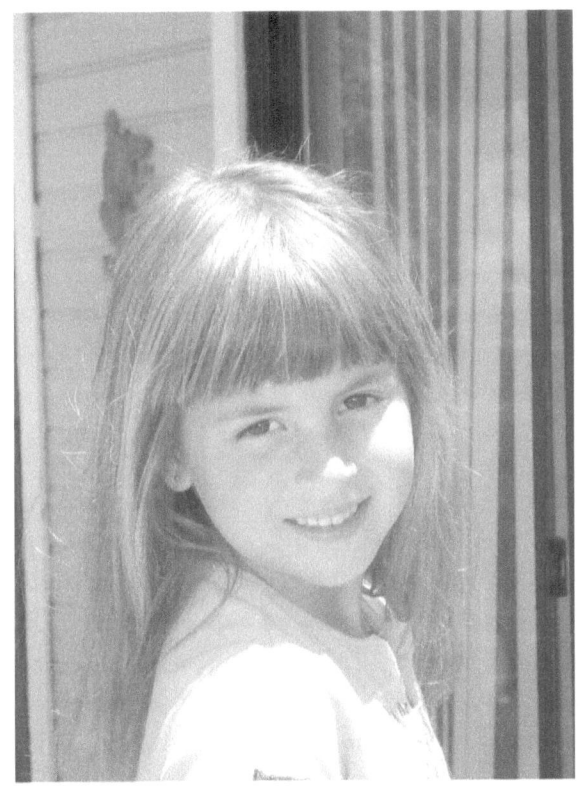

Rebecca Nicole Burton

4

FIGHTING MY FEARS

After my first surgery, where they removed the tumor and lump, the wait for results was ridiculous. I honestly believe that one of the things most difficult for me was the waiting process for results of each operation. At times I had to wait almost three weeks without knowing the gravity of my illness, and this is when my mind played with me, desperation owned me. I wanted to know everything all at once.

I tried to do something I thought was productive. I started calling the doctor's office so they'd know I was anxiously waiting for my results. They told me they'd call the next day and if they didn't, I would call them again. (Never wait for them to call you, you call and let them know how anxious you are). Finally, and with much difficulty, I understood and learned that one should have patience. Now I know that they're doing their job and I am not the only sick person in the world.

The day of the results was a day when reality set in. I felt very optimistic, very positive of the results I was about to receive, and for that reason, I decided to go alone. (Never go to the doctor alone especially if they're going to give your final results). I waited for over half an hour to speak with the doctor, half an hour that turned into an eternity. Finally in the doctor's office, he examined my surgical scar, we even told jokes, everything seem to go perfectly until he looked at me and said: "I have the results in my hand and the truth is you have breast cancer".

I didn't know what to say, I felt everything cloud up in my head and all I could say was "Am I going to die?" He said, "He hoped not" and kept talking but I didn't hear, see or feel. Finally the doctor noticed and all I could say was: "Okay, I am going home now to cry a little and you call me to let me know what steps we are to take". I stood up, went to my car and I think that was when I understood what was happening and what awaited me.

When I arrived home I hugged my mother who, thank God, was visiting from Venezuela. I cried for 3 days straight. I called my husband, we were separated at that time, and told him the bad news. He asked me to come back home, I didn't know what to do, all my feelings were mixed up and I wasn't sure that he wanted me back because he loved me or was feeling sorry for me. I moved back home anyhow. As fate would have it, three days later he was promoted and moved three hours away from me and his daughter. He would come home every weekend to help as much as he could. I would go to sleep every night praying that I would wake up the next morning from a nightmare. I was completely depressed.

One never dreams that such things can happen to you, we hear about a neighbor, a friend, or a friend of a friend, but to you? Never! Then I understood and asked myself, "why not me? I am not special, I'm the same as the others", and I knelt and said to God: "You chose me to endure this trial and I promise you that I won't question you, I will do my best to get through this and give you what you wish to see in me, only give me time to understand and put things in order. Protect me and help me be brave in what awaits me."

At times I think many of us haven't known how to appreciate life, that we're wasting time talking about others for good or bad, or what they'll say, blaming others, we become frivolous, but when we hear of someone close who is ill we become more human, we reach out to God, we see everyone as equals, we live each day better, sum up and learn to look at things differently. That is something positive, perhaps maybe that's why God chose me, because he probably wants everyone who is around me to be closer so that they might see life as I do today. If you try to extract the positive from what you perceive as a negative you will look at life in a different light. I will give you small examples of how I look at life. When I used to wake up in the morning and saw through the window that it was raining I would get out of sorts because I had to get my umbrella out, or maybe because I just had my hair done at the salon or because I washed the car yesterday, now I'm happy to see the rain because our animals, our varieties of fruits and vegetables are receiving the precious gift of water. Another example, before when I'd get a headache, I'd get grumpy, now I'm happy of course while taking an aspirin, but why do I enjoy it? It means I'm alive, that my body functions and I'm still a part of this life.

When I finished praying and speaking to God, I remember sleeping much better that night and I could see things a little better. Then I got out of bed on the fourth day and said to myself: "I'm so afraid" but I knew I had to do something about it, the only way to conquer fear is to educate oneself, soak up the problem, involve yourself as much as you can. Do you know why? Because it is your body and the decision to do what's necessary is yours.

I took action and my first step was going to the library. I searched for every book about Breast Cancer. At home I read and re-read all the books, I also started to call people who had had breast cancer, asking questions, although some may have seemed absurd. I took charge of my illness, I was preparing myself for my next visit with the doctor because they weren't going to catch me off-guard. That for me was the most important thing, taking control and not just because I have this illness but because that's how your life should be, to know exactly what you want and if you don't know what it is yet, focus on yourself, to have a peaceful life. I asked my doctor why she thought I had contracted Breast Cancer especially since there is no history in my family, and she asked me if lately I had suffered a stressful situation. Clearly, I was going through a separation from my husband at that time. I was alone with my Daughter in an apartment. Thank God all was well economically, but I had never lived alone, and it had to happen with my Daughter. I learned how to pay bills, which is a good thing. I didn't have any of my family for support, living in a foreign country where I didn't know how the system works. I lost most of my friends because of my separation. I was fearful that I wouldn't be able to make it on my own. I felt very lonely and insecure. So, yes, I was going through a most stressful time. The Doctor told me she thought that stress is a big factor when it comes to our health and I am going to explain why. Our immune system needs energy and when we are stressed we waste or expend too much of that energy, most of all mental, and so our immune system is weakened and allows any kind of illness to afflict us. I think that is exactly what happened to me.

I have a cousin named Ester. I have learned much from her mostly because she is one who applies wisdom and life goes well for her, and that is "take life as it goes". Well, believe it or not, I have applied this also and life is much better for me. If your life is frantic try, as part of your daily routine, to have at least one hour for yourself only, take a long bath, color your nails. Maybe it is time to change your hair-do. Just take a walk, but only for you, leave the children at home and go to the bakery that is missed so much and enjoy that special pastry. Do whatever it is alone, make it your moment. Do it and you will see the difference and you'll look forward to doing it again next time. This technique is best antidepressant in the world and is proven. It will give you the opportunity to know yourself better.

Since I married, I dedicated my life to my Husband, my Daughter, my home, and my work. Don't get me wrong, it fascinates me to do so, but one, without meaning to, forgets oneself, so it's time to change your routine, plan to do something different every day, but alone and in that way you won't feel as though you're doing for everyone else, that you have and deserve your time, so emotionally you will feel better. Life is so short, enjoy it.

5

SURGERIES

They all seem endless. I had already gone through the first one when they removed the lump and the tumor and the doctor gave me the news that I had breast cancer. I prepared myself and learned all I could about the disease. Of course, as if it were rare, I had to wait quite a while for my next appointment with the doctor. Finally the day arrived, when the doctor entered, he told me and my mother that I would need another surgery as he would need to go around the area of the lump and tumor to see if I was free of the cancer. Also another surgery that same day to remove the main lymph node located in the armpit. If the event found cancerous glands in my armpit it was likely the cancer had spread to other parts of my body.

My tumor measured 2.1 cm and according to the books I had read I was in the first stages of cancer; that is to say, the beginning of my illness. The doctor needed to know how far the cancer had advanced.

The wait began again for the scheduled operation, another 2 weeks and these were agonizing weeks because my mind played with me in unimaginable ways. I tried to maintain a normal routine, work, my daughter, my house, my Mama, thank God for her. I lost so much weight that I told my mother that if I received chemotherapy I would lose even more weight. I needed her to help me gain weight, I hadn't finished telling her this when I immediately gained seven pounds. Thank you so much Mama for the delicious meals you prepared for my Daughter and Me. The days passed and I always tried from the depths of my soul to stay strong. Everyone told me I had to find strength from somewhere; take it from your Daughter, look at her, she'll carry you forward. But, you know, I didn't take it from her because each time I looked at her, the pain of thinking I might die and leave her alone, was too much to take.

I didn't know how bad the cancer had invaded my body, I didn't know if I caught it in time or if it was too late. I began to think I would abandon my daughter, it saddened me more. Don't ask me from where I drew strength. I have an idea but don't know if I drew it from there. Many people started calling me as the word got around. People from Venezuela who hadn't called in years called to lift my spirits, all my friends, all of them called, family, my mother's friends. All of them prayed for me, and I said to myself that I wasn't going to cheat anyone and if I have to die I'll die fighting until the last day of my life.

I accepted humbly all that was sent to me, but one thing I can say, I didn't want to die and the sole act of thinking it made me feel as though I was already dying.

On the day of my surgery, according to the books I had read, if they found cancerous cells in my breast where I found the lump and tumor and they were extensive, the Doctor would need to remove my breast. In the event they were not extensive, the doctor would only remove the rest of the cells. I told myself if they remove my breast, it'll be better because in that way the cancer will not return, and also I could get bigger breasts! What worried me more was if the Doctor found cancer cells in my armpit there was a possibility they had spread to my vital organs.

The books I read, which were my only allies said that after the operation I'd have under my arm a drainage tube, that was because they found cancer cells, and if I'd come out without the drainage tube it was because it was negative.

Before the surgery, the doctors injected a radioactive substance in my left breast (where the cancer was found), this substance illuminates all the glands under my armpit and in this manner the doctor can easily identify the specific gland to be taken and analyzed. After waiting about 2 hours, I developed a fever, I don't know if it was due to the injection or the extreme nervousness, so the anesthesiologist did not want the surgery to proceed. I wanted it to be over as soon as possible.

My doctor, the anesthesiologist, my mom and I were talking about the situation. The anesthesiologist put a thermometer for the third time in my mouth, but this time I pretended to place it under my tongue so that my fever would not register. I wanted that surgery. If the doctor postponed the surgery it meant I'd have another 2 weeks of agonizing wait. Finally, the doctor said to the anesthesiologist that he couldn't wait. They didn't know how sick I was, so they took me to the operating room. On awakening in recovery, the first thing I did was touch under my arm to see if I felt the drainage tube, everything was bandaged but I didn't feel the drain. Of course, I was happy. When my husband, Mama and Mother-in-Law came in, they told me the doctor had said that everything looked good although the pathologist is the one with the final word, so guess what we had to do? Wait for the results.

When I arrived at home, I looked in the mirror and saw only bandages and when I touched them I felt nothing. I thought they had removed my breast and no one wanted to tell me, the doctor said not to remove the bandages until my next appointment, my desperation and curiosity were such that I didn't follow his orders and I took only the part of my bandage to see if my breast was still there. Before doing so, I hesitated and tried to imagine myself without a breast. That image was awful but it was something I had to do to prepare myself if only a little. Finally, after many false starts, due to fear, I removed the bandage. Thank God there was just a scar, I still had my breast. I told God "okay up 'til now everything seems to be going fine, please don't abandon me during this journey because it's just starting and I need you for the long process". Truly, during this time I got closer to God.

6

FINAL RESULTS

Finally after waiting for my next appointment, where the doctor was to give me the final results, my sister Reveca travelled from Oregon solely to be with me the day of the appointment. Don't ever go alone to hear such important news, I thank you so much sister.

For the results my mother, my sister and my husband Trace all came with me. Thank God we didn't have to wait long and when the doctor came in, he gave me a big hug, I didn't know the meaning of that hug, is he hugging me because it is too late or because I am okay? Finally he gave me a look and told me they found no sign of cancer in the breast or my lymph nodes.

You have no idea how happy I felt. I cannot describe the feeling. But then the doctor said to me that he was sending me to an oncologist anyway to prevent a recurrence of the cancer in either breast. I asked him how we could prevent a recurrence and he said the word I feared most in all the world, that word was ... CHEMOTHERAPY.

To my astonishment and pride, I heard myself saying to the doctor, "if it had to be done I am totally prepared," the most important thing is that I am going to be fine. Without being convinced, I along with my mom and Reveca set out to celebrate. I remember clearly the night before my final consultation, I was in my room and, as always, I lit a candle for my father, I asked him to send me strength to deal with whatever the results might be. I told him I would be most grateful if he would put in a good word for me to The Almighty. I also asked to stay close to me during my ordeal and although I love him very much, I'm not quite ready to be reunited with him. I'm quite satisfied with our present means of communication and I know he is aware of my needs, pains and hopes.

After our celebration, Reveca, Mama and I returned home to lie down in the living room and watch TV and that moment I turned my head to the left and saw the photograph of my father that I keep on the mantel and he was looking at me roguishly with that look that, was so familiar and I knew immediately what he was conveying. I cried a little and was so grateful to him for being "with" me. I love you so much Papa, one day we'll meet again but it's a bit too soon for this lady.

When do we begin? I remember the peace I felt inside, but that feeling didn't last too long, my mind began again to play with me. I kept thinking about the chemotherapy, my hair, the fatigue, and all the changes in general. It was to be a new and unknown step that I was to come to know. You experience tremendous anxiety because you find yourself in a situation that is completely out of your control. It's out of your hands, where anguish is your closest friend and try as you may you cannot change it. You know full well that the worst is over finding out the grade of your illness, looking at your daughter and asking yourself what will happen to her if I'm gone? Will she remember me.? The confusion was so overwhelming, so many things come to mind at once that you lose control, you want to cry, to die and get it over with.

Here is where I entered again and told myself "The battle is not won without a fight!" so I went back to the library where at this point everybody knew me, and I soaked up all the information on the types of chemotherapy, it's effects and duration. After learning all this I felt calmer, I was taking action again for my life. Today, I understand that these thoughts are normal when you go through the process of acceptance. You must fight, you have to fight.

Because I had no sign of cancer in my body, the chemotherapy would be preventative or less strong and perhaps my hair wouldn't fall out. I told myself that it was just hair. It'll grow back, maybe with different color and texture. I tried every which way to see the positive side but I never forgot my sister Soraya's words "it's easy to say, but to live it is another story." How right you were sister with those words. I also read that with chemotherapy I was to experience nausea and vomiting, but I know that there are many anti-nausea tablets and that was reassuring. Then there was fatigue, I said to myself, I have no problem taking a good siesta so that's okay. I also read that during this time you possibly experience loss of memory, given that I don't have a great memory anyway, don't despair I said, it'll pass. I looked at the situation superficially, on the surface because truly I wanted it that way, but if we always got what we wanted, this world would not be this world.

7

GETTING TO KNOW MY ONCOLOGIST

After waiting almost two weeks to meet my new doctor, her name is Doctor Deborah Villa: my sister, mother, husband and I, finally met her. I expected someone completely different, she was smaller and thinner than I and you could see that she was cultured and very well educated, a very sweet person. I felt extremely at ease with her from the first day. She sat in front of me and asked a series of questions, including my family history, how many children I had, where I lived and so forth. She showed much interest in my case. First she explained, using sketches, my situation and how to proceed. My sister Reveca acted as my secretary writing every word, my "rurita" as I call her, as always, prepare for everything. Dr. Villa explained that my cancer, sadly, was an aggressive type and as a consequence they would need and aggressive form of chemotherapy. She also explained that I would need an examination, MRI, to determine any cancerous cells in my body. This gives a head-to-toe picture. She explained the manner in which the chemotherapy was going to affect my body, including hair loss, fatigue, nausea, vomiting, infertility, difficulty remembering things and menopause, temporary or permanent depending on how my body tolerated it. I began laughing and told her I'd bet I wouldn't suffer any of the beforementioned symptoms, but I would suffer from the hot flashes of menopause. She said to stay away from sick people and that my immune system would be affected. I looked at her straight in the eye and told her I was ready.

For the first two months of my chemotherapy, every two weeks consisted of two drugs combined ADRYAMICIN and CITOXIN. After the first two months of these drugs, I would receive two consecutive months, every two weeks, of one drug TAXOL. That's a total of four months of chemotherapy. After that, she would refer me to a radiologist to finalize my treatment.

I left the consultation very satisfied with my doctor's attitude. It's very important that you feel comfortable and satisfied with your doctors. If, on the contrary you don't have complete confidence, stay calm, you have time to search out other doctors who will make you feel better. Remember it's your body, your decision.

-The MRI

Even though I was calm about the results, the fact that the doctor had ordered that type of examination was probably because she suspected something or knew something that I didn't know. The nervousness returned because those tests don't lie. The night before the MRI, I had to drink a radioactive liquid made with sugar (cancerous cells are attracted to sugar) and the day of the MRI I had to drink another one. I recall that night I didn't sleep at all, nerves, desperation, loneliness, didn't let me think clearly, it was a long night.

Finally, the day arrived and I was treated wonderfully at the doctor's office. I began to prepare myself for the ordeal. It would be simple but took a long time. I got an unbearable headache. I knew it was nervousness and not having slept the night before. The next day at the oncologist office the doctor told me that there were no visible cancer and if there should be even the smallest cancer cell the chemotherapy would eliminate it. Thank God for this news. For the first time in months I slept like a baby.

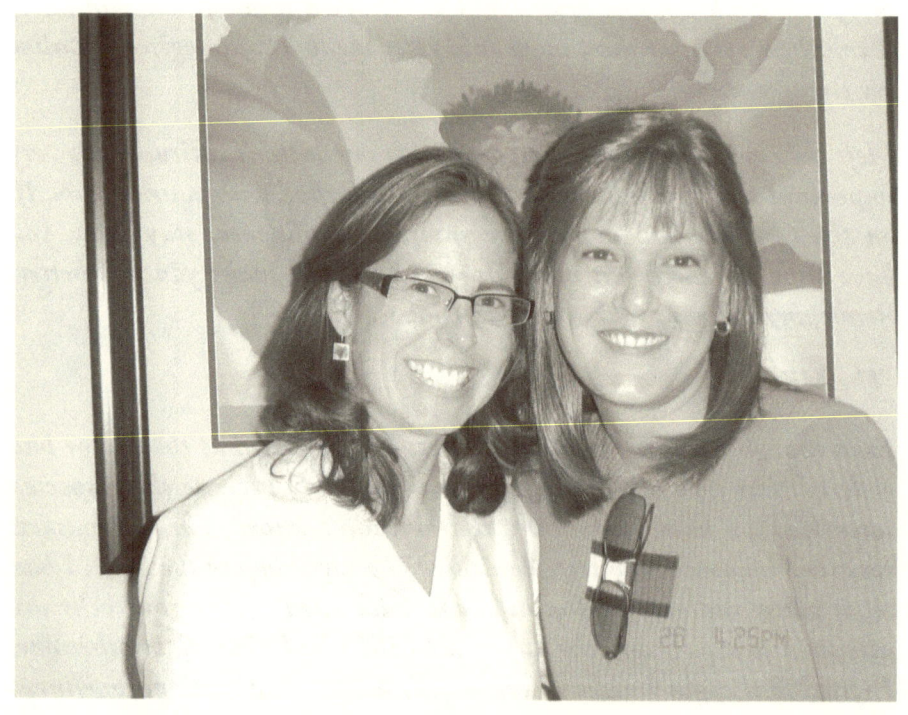

My Doctor Deborah Villa and I

8

SIGNIFICANCE OF CHEMOTHERAPHY

It is a treatment for cancer based on toxic drugs. These drugs are designed to find and destroy cancerous cells. Side effects occur because healthy cells are also destroyed. The drugs must be toxic to be effective, but those used to fight breast cancer are less harmful. In women who still have menstrual periods they administer commonly a combination of three drugs, as they did in my case.

The types of drugs depend on the level found in the cancer. I am level one, that is to say, beginning stage. Chemotherapy can be administered in different ways:

-To cure the cancer when it is thought the patient is free of any evidence of cancer cells.

-To control the cancer, this prevents the return of the disease, controlling the growth and killing cells that may have spread to other organs away from the original tumor.

-To alleviate the symptoms cancer may cause, such as pain and discomfort. It can help the patient live a more comfortable life.

Today, chemo is much easier to tolerate than in previous years. It is important to understand that in the organs in which the cells do not divide rapidly such as the liver and kidneys, it is rare that they are affected by chemo.

8.1 HOW CHEMOTHERAPY AFFECTS CELLS

The body produces cells in the bone marrow and this produces platelets, red cells and white cells. Chemotherapy interferes with the ability of the bone marrow to make cells in the blood. During chemo, it is necessary to count the number of platelets, red and white cells in the blood and if these are found to be low or irregular the chemo should be suspended until they returned to normal.

8.2 TYPES OF BLOOD CELLS

-Platelets: they help control excessive bleeding and bruising.

-Red Cells: Provide oxygen to the body trough the veins. When these cells are low in count it is called anemia and this can cause fatigue, shortness of breath or dizziness.

-White Cells: Control infections in the body. When these cells are low it is called neutropenia, which makes it difficult to control infections.

8.3 WHEN CELLS ARE FOUND TO BE LOW

When the cells in our body are found to be low, infection, fatigue, bleeding or more serious complications may occur. It is important to monitor and control the level of these cells to reduce side effects and delay the chemotherapy.

Reducing or delaying chemo can in some cases cause the treatment to be less effective, but maintaining the cells at a healthy level is vitally important to assure that your treatment be timely so as to obtain best results, so that the cells will remain at a healthy level. It is also important that you are properly nourished even though your appetite is poor. Eating small portions every three hours may be tolerated better than a normal meal.

9

TREATMENTS

The treatment you will receive depends on your diagnosis. You will have at least one surgery and subsequently a combination of chemo, radiation or hormone treatments. Not all women with breast cancer receive the same treatment. Surgery that saves part of the breast is called conservative. Mastectomy is when the breast is removed completely. Pregnant women need not terminate the pregnancy but in some cases it is advisable to have the baby early. The type of treatment pregnant women receive depends on the time of pregnancy, the size of the tumor and the characteristics of the tumor.

Sometimes chemo is the only treatment the patient may receive, however, chemo is used additionally with surgery, radiation and biological therapy to:

-bind the tumor before surgery or radiation.

-Help destroy any cancerous cells that remained in the system after surgery or radiation.

-Assure that the radiation and therapy work better, more effectively.

-Help destroy the return of the cancer or if it has spread to other parts of the body from the original source.

10

MY FIRST CHEMOTHERAPY

Before I started my chemotherapy, the first thing I did was to order a wig (it's the first thing you should do so the change won't be so drastic.) I remember going to the wig store with my sister Reveca and my Mom to find a wig for me, and when I entered the store there were wigs everywhere. They were beautiful, different colors and sizes and I started trying them on one after another one. At first, it was fun looking at myself in the mirror and laughing at all of them and it seemed that none of them suited me and all of a sudden what had seemed fun turned to frustration. I broke down and cried. I never imagined myself in a situation such as this. I then realized that this was no joke, this was being done out of necessity. The store clerk calmed me down and little by little she showed me more wigs one after another and made suggestions that were helpful. Finally, we ordered a wig that was the same color as mine and longer than my own hair. When it arrived, I was going to take it to my hair stylist who would cut it to my own style.

The final result was incredible! My wig was an exact replica of my own natural hair. Now I was ready for my first chemo treatment. The doctor prescribed the pills to avoid nausea and vomiting with the instructions included. When I arrived at the doctor's office, I remember looking around and seeing only older people there to receive chemotherapy and I was the youngest and that made me sad and lonely. I wanted to run away. I felt sorry for myself. For a moment, I thought that it wasn't fair, but I tried to stay calm and keep telling myself that I wasn't the only one in this world. I was very scared and I didn't feel strong at all. The nurses took me to a room with three chairs, two reclining and one for the person accompanying me. A music system played relaxing tunes and behind the chairs were all kinds of books to read, there were plants, lots of blankets, on the walls were lovely paintings. What caught my attention, however, was a goldfish bowl with just one little fish who was as lonely as I was. The room was very comforting nonetheless.

I met my charming nurse, her name is Phya, she began explaining the process. First, she inserted a needle in my vein and start giving me the medication for the nausea. She had trouble finding my vein, so on my next treatment I would need a catheter, a device placed by general surgery under the skin, in the upper part of the right side of my breast where the major vein connects and makes the chemotherapy much easier and faster. Thank God for modern technology. After the medication for the nausea was placed in my system, the nurse inserted the toxic drugs, Adryamicin and Citoxin. I felt very good at that point and even spoke to my mother and the nurses and I even drank a cup of coffee. To be sure, I felt a little drowsy due to the effects of the anti-nausea drugs. After an hour and a half the toxic drugs were finally in my system, but I felt fine and when Mama and I returned home we sat down to lunch. My daughter was to stay with my mother-in-law in case I got sick and I didn't want her to see me in that condition. I will always remember that day, after we ate lunch, I remember the look in my mom's eyes, she insisted very much for me to eat and I did. I was happy that I wasn't feeling sick, but she kept looking at me and took me to my bed, and told me that I needed to rest. I know now that she totally knew what was coming. We got home around 1;00pm and at 3:00pm I felt as though I was dying.

I felt a heat throughout my entire body and I began to vomit again and again. My headache was so intense that I thought my scalp was burning and that's when I knew my hair would fall out. My mom put an ice pack on my head and the ice would melt in less than an hour. It was so painful that at one point I took my mom's hand and told her that I know now what my father had gone through. The only thing I could think of was that I have seven more treatments to go. I wanted to die. I didn't think I'd make it through the rest. I don't remember how many times I vomited and I didn't know how to stop. I took a few more pills, but it was too late, once you start vomiting, no matter what you do, it won't stop. I felt very lonely and very afraid, I wanted to give up.

The next day, I had to see the doctor to get an IV bag because I was so dehydrated due to all the vomiting, The also gave me morphine to ease the pain, and on top of that, they gave me a shot of Neulasta to raise my white blood cells. I will get the Neulasta a day after every treatment. The effects of chemo last three days, in my case five days, and after the treatment I felt as though I had a terrible sun burn, my skin even started to peel. That's how my body reacted. It hurt when I was touched—even my bones ached; I thought they would break. I understood why people fear that word "chemo". I was completely drugged on the medicine and my poor mother was going through the same experience as she suffered with my father and it almost killed me just seeing the suffering on her face, for that reason I drew all the strength possible and got out of bed. I tried to live a normal life again. A week after my treatment, I went to see my doctor again and she couldn't believe what I had gone through, she said generally people don't suffer so, that only 4 % of patients get such headaches. I also had acute sinusitis and I thought I was getting sick and the first thing she told me was to try and stay well and to stay away from sick people or the chemo would have to be delayed.

When I told her about my sinusitis, she said it was unusual but about 3% of patients were affected, I started to laugh and stopped asking questions about my symptoms in case that number got to 1%. My doctor never thought the reaction would be so severe and said we'd have to make adjustments next time, and I told her, "the only way possible is to put me to sleep for three days," I began to laugh again and, to my surprise, she said they could do that. I went home in a good mood, thinking that the next treatment would be much better.

11

PHYSICAL CHANGES

My doctor told me that my hair would begin falling out after my second chemo, but after the way my skin felt after the first time I didn't think I'd have any hair for my second treatment. That's how it turned out. One day, I was in the shower and I noticed how much hair remained in my hand. I tried not to touch it and I went days without combing it, but it was inevitable and sad to try to hold on to something that it was going to happen no matter what.

It was Mother's Day that I decided to shave my head. I wanted to involve my family in the process so there would be no shock, so I looked at my daughter and told her that this day I was going to allow her to do something only once. She looked at me and asked me what it was. I told her today you are going to be my personal hair stylist so get ready to cut my hair. I'll never forget that day, I sat in the chair, my daughter was behind me playing with my hair, pieces were flying everywhere and the look on my daughter's face was indescribable, she was having fun, and while she was laughing, I cried, but she never saw me.

My sister Soraya was right, the moment when reality set in, was this time, and it hurt. When my daughter got tired, I let my husband shave my head completely. My mother wasn't there, obviously, she did not want to participate in the process. When I felt my head, and didn't feel a single hair, I went to look for my mother, I closed the door to her bedroom and we cried together for a long time. When I came out of her room, I went straight to put on my new wig, but as it was all so new to me, I didn't know how to style it and I was even afraid to go outside for fear it would fly away! I began buying hats of all kinds, sporty, elegant, but everyone told me I didn't need them as my wig looked so natural. I still felt very self-conscious.

When I went out for the first time wearing my wig, I felt as though everyone was looking at me and knew what was happening to me. Of course this is a normal reaction nowadays. I had to regain my identity, learn to accept myself and not retreat into myself. When this adjustment period was past, I would care very little what people thought.

It took a month to learn to style and maintain the wig and I even tried new hairdos and eventually I put the hats away as they only made me feel hotter. Little by little my confidence returned and everything got easier. In the shower, I didn't have to worry about washing my hair or shaving, I could shower in five minutes. I learned to make up my face to better emphasize my eyes. I felt more beautiful than ever because it was better to look your best than sickly. I'll tell you the truth, there were times that I couldn't get out of bed, but my daughter would kiss my bald head every morning and tell me I am her favorite mom, of course I'm her only one, and I made each day the best one of my life.

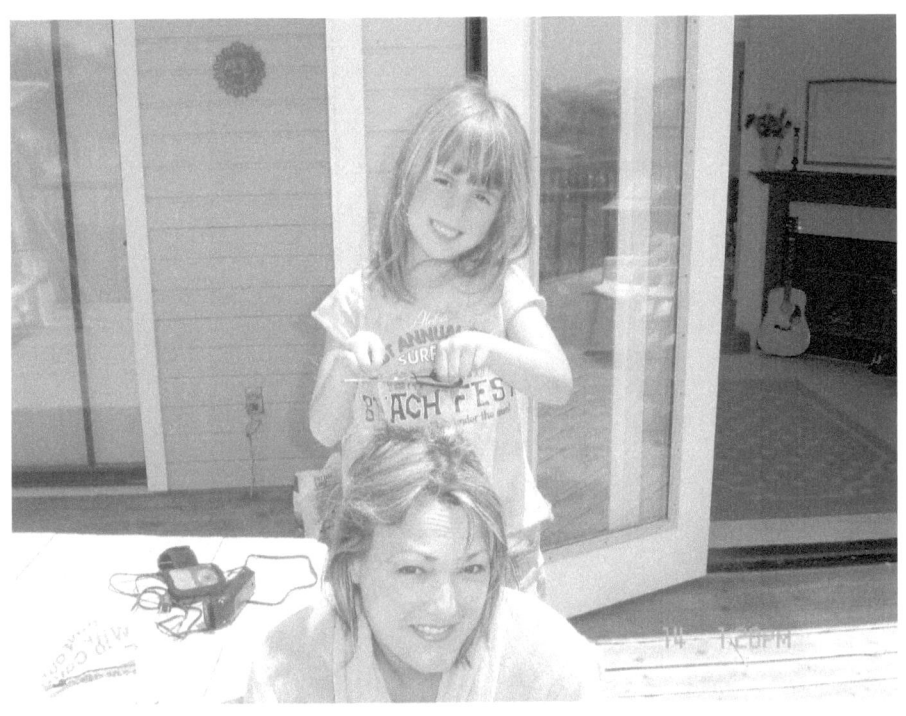

My daughter cutting my hair

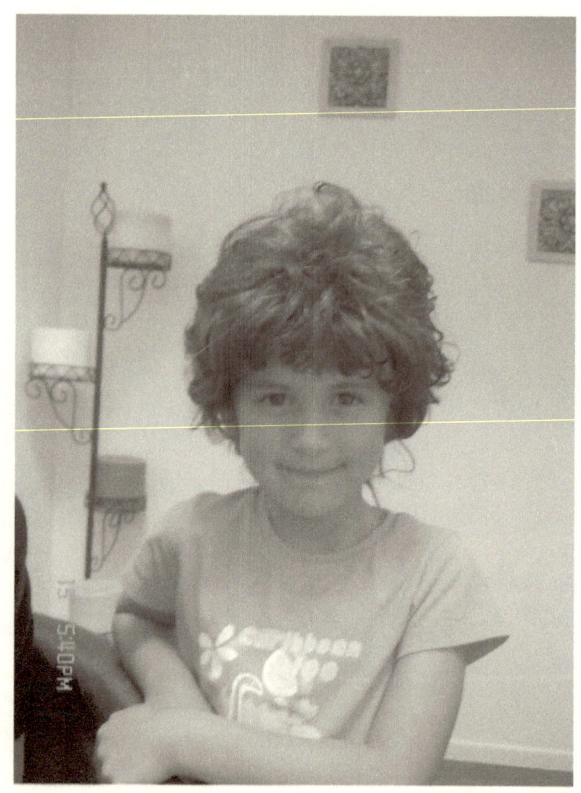

My daughter wearing one of my wigs

12

MY SECOND CHEMOTHERAPY

As part of my routine, I was preparing myself for my second chemother-
apy, having blood tests, consultation with my doctor and making sure I
followed all instructions so that nothing would go wrong this time. My
cousin Alicia was visiting from Miami helping my Mama, she stayed
for two weeks and among the experiences we shared was one night we
decided to go out and party and listen to one of my favorite band and
have a few drinks. We both dressed up and looked beautiful and I got
my wig and a spectacular hat. We attracted a lot of attention, when we
arrived, and my cousin met a charming bald young man. We were hav-
ing a good time, when suddenly a young man approached me and
asked me what that fellow was doing talking to my cousin. He said,
"He is ugly" and furthermore, "bald"! I was tempted to remove my wig
and tell him that in that case, he shouldn't have been talking to me.
Life, in that moment, showed me that one should never judge another
person by their appearance, because you never know. My cousin and I
had fun and she helped me so much. It calmed me somewhat to know
that she would stay and help me and my mom emotionally.

I don't deny that I feared a repeat of what happened after my first
chemo. The day I arrived, during the consultation, I spoke with the sec-
retaries, joking, laughing but then resigned, I sat in the chair. Then, I
endured the same process as before, the same nausea and vomiting
drugs, the IV bag and then the drugs. When finished, the first thing I
did on arriving home was take more nausea pills and sleeping pills. I

lay down on the bed with my pail for vomiting at my side and waited. I was nervous and scared. I felt so lonely and I kept waiting but the hours passed and nothing happened. I fell asleep and awakened. I ate, looked at my mom and told her that I couldn't believe it, I have no pain, and that's how it went for the next few days. I felt some pain in my body, the sensation of heat and burn, but nothing more. It was magic. I had my realistic nightmares. I perspired very much and contracted acute sinusitis. I also had what felt like a hangover.

I was aware that the chemicals that were killing my cells were so powerful that when I cried, which was very often, my tears were sticky. As the days passed, I noticed that my nails were growing very fast and my skin was so smooth. Of course the chemo was killing new and old cells and all the cells that were reproducing were new cells. My complexion and everything that was growing was pretty much virgin. You are aware that everything has a positive side, if you believe it.

Three days after my chemo, I felt perfectly fine. My mom, my daughter and I, decided to go to the park. We even went for walks. I still felt dizzy most of the times, but this was definitely my best chemo. I was still keeping my weight thanks to my mom. I also took advantage of feeling so good, that I played with my daughter as much as I could.

We took a trip to where my husband lived. I wanted to get out of my house. Rebecca enjoyed the trip and I have to admit that my mom and I enjoyed it, too. I remember that we heard an ice cream truck, which is very unusual. My mom, Rebecca and I raced out the door to get ice cream and half way there I remembered I had forgotten to put on my wig! Of course, when I became aware of that fact, I ran into the house laughing so hard. Many episodes such as this have happened when I forgot my wig.

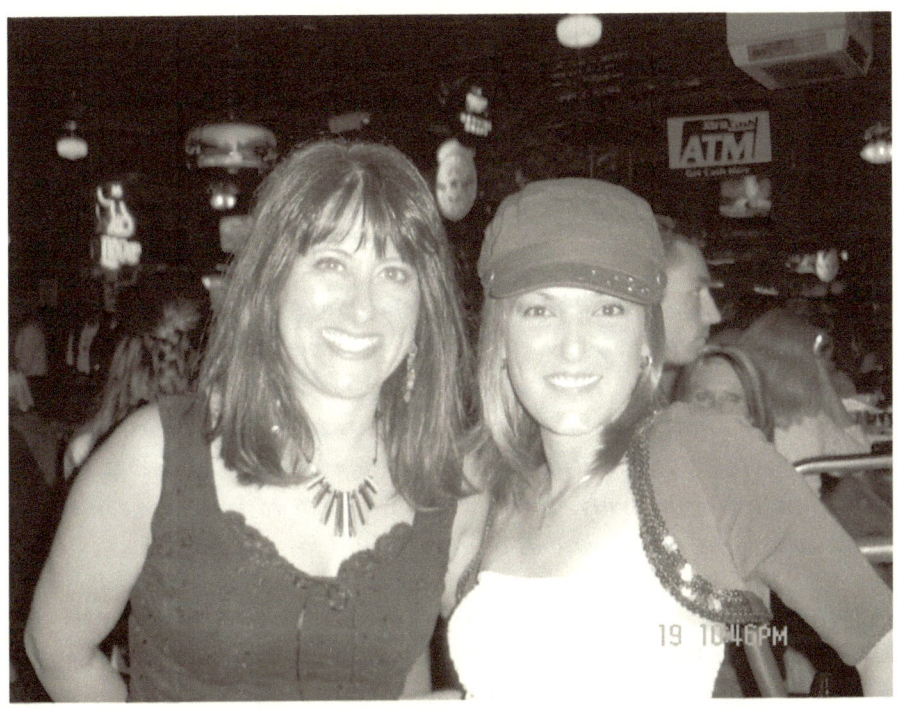

My cousin Alicia and I a day before my second quimo

13

MY THIRD CHEMOTHERAPY

I was more prepared and more confident about this chemo. I thought, my second went so well, I'm going to be positive and this one will also go well. I felt drained. My spirits were pretty low as I kept thinking I still had five more chemotherapy treatments to go. I switched methods then, so instead of counting how many more I had to have, I'd say that's one less and, truly, I only had one week to rest between treatments to try and recuperate as best as I could for the next one.

I continued to live as normal life as possible. I tried to stay busy so that the time would pass faster. But fatigue would overtake me and I'm only 36 years old! I can't imagine someone at age 70 (there were many that I saw) but I'll always be me and I'd always be cheerful and laugh with everyone and I tried not to talk about my situation so as not to tire anyone, especially those who would ask "how are you?" I'd answer "marvelous" and the more I'd say it the more I believed it, although, the main person and only one who accompanied me in my true suffering was my Mama.

The day before my chemo, I tried to meditate and do my breathing exercises to alleviate my anxiety somewhat. My daughter would always go to my in-laws the day before my chemo to spend at least two days with them. That night I spent for me, I went out to spend a good time with a very special friend, someone that was always there every time I called, a friend that was always open to listen and made me feel good.

When I got home, I found myself very relaxed and took a long bath. I washed my wig so that it would shine the next day. I chose the clothes I'd wear, always matching them with my hat. I prepared my carrot, orange and beet juice cocktail which I began drinking since I learned I had cancer and finishing the evening with a good, humorous book to read. The next day came with the usual routine, the consultation office, my nurse Phya and the needle again in my chest where the Chemo would go. This time, I slept throughout the entire process, due to the many drugs they had given me. Most of the time, I didn't even know where I was.

I remember, after I arrived home after the second chemotherapy, my mom and cousin Alicia were in the kitchen. I passed by them in my lingerie and told them to hurry up as we were going to be late, grabbed my purse and I was at the door when they guided me back to bed. After my third chemo, I was looking for something in my bedroom that was making so much noise that I thought I was going crazy. My mom was right next to me, and she never heard anything. That was part of the drugs' effects, but of course, I don't remember a thing.

My mom started to worry that I'd leave the house without being aware of it. So, from the first day of chemo, she slept with me. I always ate what my mom prepared for me. This time, I felt the chemo stronger in my body even though I slept for three days. I was already feeling the tiredness and it took more days to recuperate almost completely. I didn't feel up to going out. I rarely went to work. I started to get depressed. I cried a lot especially upon awakening when reality hit me. I knew it was not just a bad dream and it was a bigger effort to start the day.

When I felt my daughter kiss my bald head and I became aware that I was not only fighting emotions but also fighting physically. I didn't get dressed anymore. I spent more time at home and being tired didn't help. I cried so much. I didn't feel love. I was very lonely. I knew that I must not fall into this state of depression. I had a long way to go and I would make it worse if I gave in to death. I stood up and decide to keep fighting for my life.

I wanted to give up so many times. I told myself that I had never finished what I had started. I always gave up half way. I wasn't too good at keeping promises and never took anything seriously. It's was time to prove to myself that I could fight. I promised to win and end this battle and if God permitted, I could do it. I changed my attitude and went forward. I got out of bed and saw the light of day again. I knew life was waiting for me out there and I promised myself that I was going to live.

14

MY FOURTH CHEMOTHERAPY

I felt more prepared for my fourth chemo and was confident that it would be as easy as the second. The same routine, blood test, doctor's appointments, all resulted well and I was happy that it was going to be the last treatment that combined the 2 drugs (Adryamicin and Citoxin), the fifth would require only one drug, (Taxol). I was ready physically, although a bit tired, but I noticed that the more I slept the more tired I became, so I tried sleeping less. I also noticed that I was starting to forget things and I had trouble focusing on making decisions. My menstrual period had stopped after the second chemo, but I knew this was temporary and the method by which the chemo was administered would make me more tired. I was ready. I received my fourth dose, and this time I noticed that the nurse gave me all the mixed drugs at the same time. So, I asked her why. I always asked a lot of questions. She said that another patient had the drugs administered in that manner and the effects were more favorable for her. I didn't say anything but on arriving home I felt very, very sick, not as bad as the first time, but I vomited so many times that I can't even remember. I was nauseated for nine days. I ate and threw up, I lost 7 pounds in 8 days and I couldn't keep anything in my stomach.

The exhaustion and fatigue had turned into my allies. I was beginning to lose my strength which meant, that recuperation would take longer each time. I lost what little patience I had left, everything bothered me. I even purposely broke things around the house. Uselessness took over, it was uncontrollable the desperation that I felt. Nothing helped relieve the nausea and now everything that my Mom prepared for me was repugnant.

When you find yourself in that situation, you sink, cry and you just know that you'll never be normal and you'll live in constant fear that your cancer will return. You see other people laughing, enjoying the day seeming to not having a care in the world. So I felt pain and anger at the same time. I was uncomfortable with the doctor because if, as she said, I was making progress, why change the method of administering the drugs? I felt as though they have used me. I started to live my daily life again, trying to keep busy as best I could. I tried to get to work as soon as I felt better always thinking, one less treatment, soon it'll be easier, the worst is over.

I tried to see things a little bit better although most of the times I was weak. I remember one morning I awoke and decided to go out with my mother and Rebecca to a lovely outdoor spot where we could feed the animals, buy fresh vegetables grown there and stroll around and have a picnic with my family. The ice cream sold there is the best I've ever had in my life. When we arrived, my mom and daughter were walking hurriedly. I tried to keep with them but couldn't. I felt very tired and the sun was making me feel weaker. My legs got so that they barely responded to my efforts to keep up, and I tried so hard to keep walking but I felt dizzy. So, sadly and with tears in my eyes, I had to find a shade tree and wait and cool off. Thanks to my mom again for making sure my daughter could enjoy herself.

We all had ice cream and they sat down under the shade tree with me but sadly, I couldn't enjoy it as the chemo gives a metallic taste to everything and I couldn't enjoy food at all. I always told myself that tomorrow would be better than today. I said this a thousand times: "I must fight, I must get up, I can't feel sorry for myself", and that's how I continued my journey that didn't seem quite so long anymore.

15

MY FIFTH CHEMOTHERAPY

We all thought this one would be a breeze. Just one drug and, supposedly, the only effects would be nausea and pain in the bones, especially in the joints. It sounded good to me since I had suffered so much after the previous treatments. This would be easy. We even made plans for my mom to visit my sister Reveca in Oregon. My discomfort should only last for two days and would be eased taking ibuprofen. I thought that since they'd only send me home with one little pill, it meant that it couldn't be anything serious. I met a woman there who was receiving that drug and she said she was fine.

I was calm and happy and thought only three treatments after this. When I arrived at the doctor's I asked her again about the effects I would have. She reconfirmed their benefits and said "Believe me, this time you're going to be fine", I asked the doctor if this would be a good time for my mother to leave for a visit to Oregon and she said this would be the perfect time for her to go. Mama decided to postponed the trip, until she could assure herself that I was going to be fine. If everything went well she'd go as planned. In a way I was glad she was to go. It didn't seem fair that she was living with such pain and I really wanted her to enjoy a vacation. I felt guilty for making her suffer, days before my chemo's she'd get so nervous her blood pressure would climb and I don't think it ever came down. Naturally, deep inside, I didn't want her to go, there's no one like a mother to take care of you. Where you don't care if she sees you vomiting, or bald, or without makeup or clothes or crying, but I couldn't be selfish, not with my mother.

41

The day arrived, and my mom and I decided to take breakfast to the secretaries, doctors and, of course, us. The process began and I was connected the IV bag and we were all in the room talking and laughing. After an hour, the IV was removed and it was time to administer the new drug Taxol. Everything seemed to be going as planned, we even decided to eat breakfast. As I began eating and talking to my Mom, all of the sudden I felt an intense heat that went completely throughout my body. I stopped eating and I started to pay attention to the changes in my body. I began to feel such an intense pain in my stomach that everything in my mouth came out. I told my mom that something was wrong and to call the nurse. While my mom was doing this, I felt nausea and the urge to vomit. I felt a pain in my chest that made it difficult for me to breathe. I could only wait while the nurse called for help. I felt as though I was going to die, my body felt light and calm but also in much pain. My heart was beating so hard that I heard the beats in my head. My life passed in front of me in fractions of seconds, my memories, especially my daughter. Thank God the nurse immediately yanked the bag connected to my chest and gave me an injection. When I became aware of what was happening, there were about four doctors in front of me. I relaxed immediately but the strangest thing of all was that I felt no fear, on the contrary, when I was feeling better I asked the doctor to insert the drug again. The doctor told me frankly that I could die and that I had had an allergic reaction to the drug and he could not possibly insert the drug again. They kept me there until I was completely stable. I already had drugs in my system to control the nausea and they made me feel very goofy.

I was very angry because I was half way through the process and to cancel now meant delaying the treatment. I felt it was time lost, as before every treatment I had to undergo many tests to make sure I was in proper physical condition to receive the chemo. I didn't want to delay it any longer. Finally, I understood what really happened. It would have been sad to survive the illness but have the remedy kill me. Finally, they let me go home and I was thinking "what now?" what kind of drug will I get? My mom will not leave on her trip until she knows what's going to happen. When we were talking to the doctor on call, my doctor was not there that day, he told us that there were other alternatives. In my case, he mentioned a drug that was used for women at stage four, almost metastasis. I asked him how can you use that on me since I was in stage one? He then told me that the only person to make that decision would be my doctor. That was the only thought on my mind when I arrived at home. I would imagine that it would be a very powerful drug, as it is used for advanced cancer.

I tried not to think about it and told myself that it was in God's hands now. My mom decided to go for a walk after we got home, and since I didn't get my treatment it would be safe for her to do that, and as I felt dizzy, decided to get in bed. After she had left, I decided to fix myself something to eat, some fried eggs. I forced myself to go to the kitchen, took out a frying pan, put some oil in the bottom of the pan, and when it was hot, don't ask me what I did or how it happened but my wig landed in the hot oil! I told myself that was all I needed, no chemo and now no wig. I heard how the oil burned my wig and I quickly took it out and put it in cold water. When I put it back on, there remained only half of it and the burnt smell was unbearable. I didn't say anything about it to my mom. It could have been worse. I could've burned myself because the drugs made me lose focus on things. What seemed like such a simple thing as frying eggs became difficult to accomplish.

The next day, I hurried to the wig shop and thank God I found one exactly like the one I had burned. God squeezes but doesn't strangle. Two days after that minor accident, I went to see my doctor. My mom had resigned herself to staying with me and not making the trip to see my sister Reveca as she was not going to leave me in my present condition. I told my mom calmly that maybe the doctor will stop the rest of the treatments because of the allergic reaction that I had. I said this jokingly and she said, "Yes daughter, only in your dreams."

At last, we entered the office and the first thing my doctor wanted to know was what had happened. I explained step by step every detail and truthfully that at my next chemo I would be very nervous because I didn't know how I would react. She told me calmly that she did not expect my reaction because it's very rare and it does not happen to everyone so I was to get no more chemotherapy because the other combination we could use was reserved solely for patients with advanced breast cancer and that didn't apply in my case, so her work was done and the next step was to be radiation treatment. When those were completed, we'd meet again to begin checking me every three months.

I heard her speaking but I couldn't believe it, I thought she was not telling the truth, that it was a lovely dream which I wished for every day but when I awoke it was the same nightmare. I asked her if it was true what she was telling me and she replied "YES," It wasn't worth taking the risk. She is my doctor and she knows what she's doing, she is not going to just let me go. Most doctors do not like to just dismiss patients, remember that chemo and radiation are preventative now that no cancer was found in my body.

The doctor must have thought that if there was a small amount of cancer in my body, the four chemo treatments would have eliminated it. I hugged everyone as I came out of the office. Lastly, I hugged my mom and the tears that flowed from us were not tears of sadness, anguish, suffering or pain. They were tears of joy, of knowing that my nightmare was over. I bet that was the gift from God for having shown my strength and acceptance, for learning to fight and look at life in a different light.

I will always carry this experience with me because it's not over yet. I will always live with the struggle inside. I don't know that I'll have to go through it again. I pray to God that he'll spare me that, but what I can tell you is that the experience taught me how to live.

That same night, I went out with friends to celebrate. For the first time, I felt like a normal person. I thought, no more treatments, no more surgeries or doctor's appointments, no more tests, for a while, at last my calendar would look emptier and more normal. The ill feelings were over. The physical and emotional pain were all in the past. That stage was over and now I was to enter another, an easier one: radiation.

Three weeks had passed since my final chemo, and I had dedicated myself to me and my daughter. My mom had left to Oregon and I missed her naturally, but I called her every day and thanked God she was having a good time. For the first time in months, I'd slept like a baby, without worries. Sometimes, I got up in the morning thinking I was going to be late for an appointment or I think I was due for more Chemo. I had nightmares but I knew this would all pass.

The worst was over. Now, I knew I must emphasize my health, physically and emotionally. I would try and see things calmer and be myself. As I said before, when one is ill, doctors focus more on the vulnerability of the immune system than the illness itself. It is also documented that physical and emotional stress weaken the Immune system. Studies show that colds are more common when stress is present. The majority of widows and widowers die less than two years after the death of their spouses, because stress completely weakens the immune system.

You must be yourself mentally, emotionally, spiritually and physically. To deny who you are truly ends in death. My doctor demonstrated a very important point in that, for every year you live with stress you are shortening your life by three years, according to this, she says if you do something without passion, only because it needs doing, and you are not happy doing it, you shorten your life another six years. If someone is draining your energy due to constant conflict, you are losing eight years. Adding to that, all the years you could lose due to stress and living a fictional life, you could be losing 32 years of your life. Think about it! It's more than one third of your life and all because we choose to live our life that way, instead of trying to live life realistically and discover new paths and, therefore, find the tools to challenge yourself. In that way, learn the difference of what is good and what is harmful. When you accomplish this, nothing or no one can unbalance you. I will be in that balance very soon.

16

RADIATION

Radiation is the use of high energy rays to destroy cancerous cells. It is usually used to guard against further damage after breast surgery. Sometimes, depending on the size of the tumor and other factors, Radiation therapy is used to eliminate breast cancer cells in the area, also after mastectomies (loss of the breast).

Some women receive radiation (alone or with chemo or hormone therapy) before surgery to destroy cancer cells and reduce the size of the tumor. This method is used with more success when the breast tumor is large or cannot be easily removed by surgery.

Doctor's use two types of radiation to combat breast cancer:

-External Radiation. This is done by machine. For external radiation, the patients go to a clinic or a hospital. Generally, these treatments are programmed every day of the week for several weeks.

-Internal radiation. This radiation consists of radioactive material consisting of two plastic thin tubes placed directly in the breast, this requires a hospital stay. The implants remain in place until the patient is released.

During radiotherapy, women with breast cancer often feel tired especially toward the end of the treatment and these feelings may continue after the treatment is completed. Rest is important but doctors generally suggest that all patients try to stay as active as possible.

It is also common for the skin around the treated area to become reddish, dry sensitive and feel burned. The breast may feel heavy and tight, however these discomforts will disappear in time.

When the treatment is almost over, the skin may become damp and sweaty. The bra and other kinds of clothing can irritate the skin so it is recommended that loose clothing such as cotton be worn during this time. Women should ask the doctor before using deodorants. This is temporary, though, and should return to normal after the treatment. However, it is possible that the color of your skin may be changed permanently.

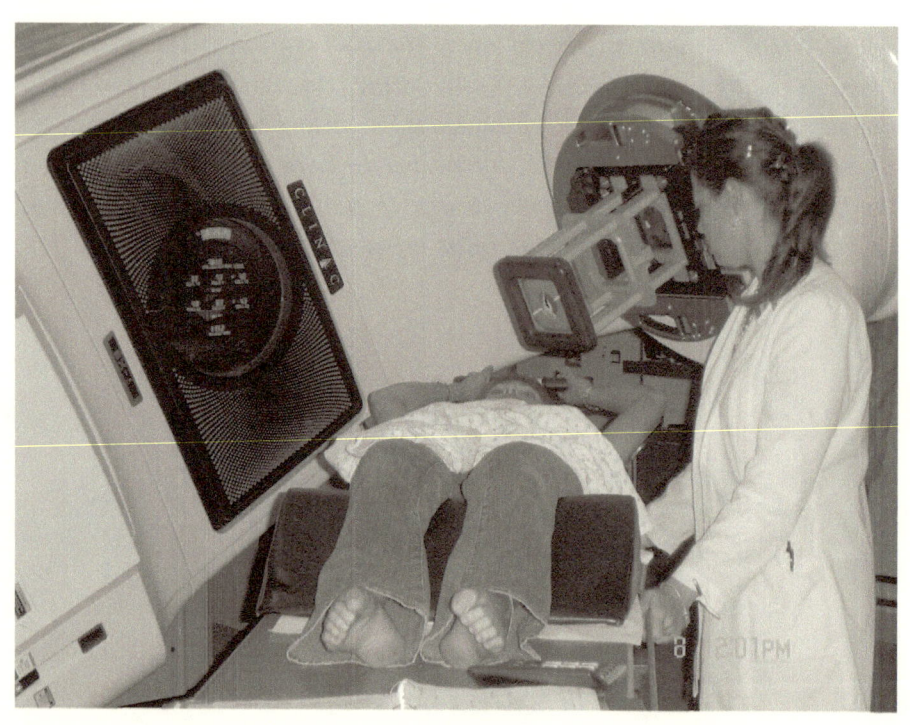

getting Radiation

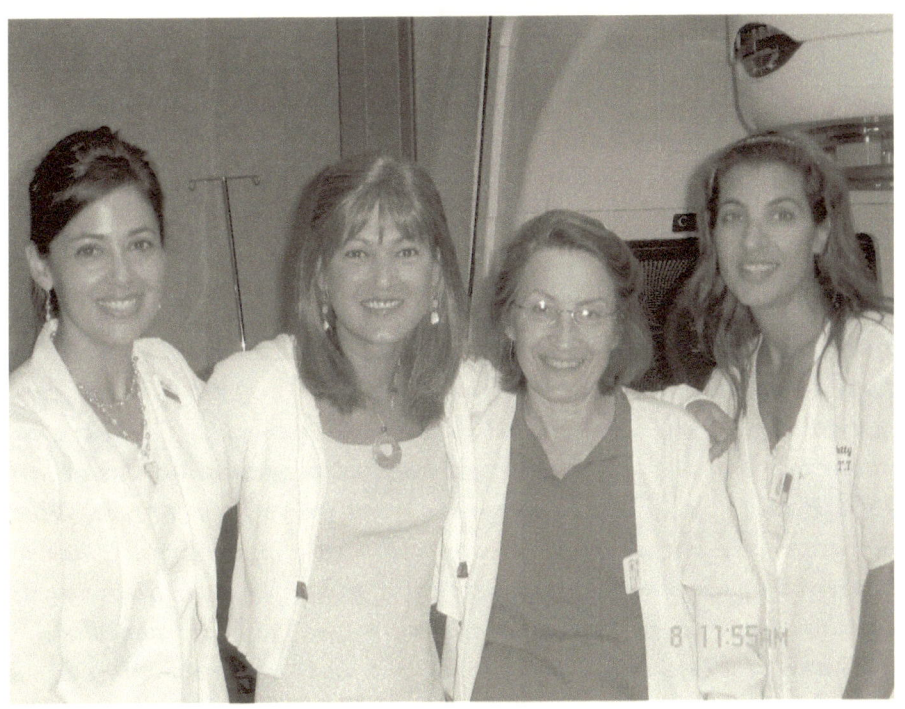

the Radiation Staff

17

PREPARING MYSELF
FOR RADIATION

When I got up that morning, I was a little nervous about this new ordeal but very calm at the same time, because I thought there was going to be no pain involved. I arrived at the treatment center very early that morning. The medical staff treated me nicely. They gave me a tour of what was to be my second home as my radiation was to last 45 days in a row. When I entered the room where I was to receive the radiation, my jaw dropped. I cannot describe my feelings. I was so impressed by the machine they were going to use for my little breast. It was immense. Then they explained what was going to take place. I remember it all exactly. They sent me to a room to disrobe and when I turned around there drawers everywhere with names for patients to place their personal clothes and jewelry. I started to look closely and all of a sudden I saw my name already on one of them.

I felt rather sad as I always wanted my name on something important and in one way or another it came true. I went directly to a table where I lay down and directly above me was that enormous machine. I was so scared, I wanted to get up and leave that room. They marked my breast and measured it. They took pictures and made marks all over my breast to determine exactly where the radiation would do its work. I remember my breast looking like a map and an intense red laser beam moved all over my breast. I was not allowed to move an inch so I just kept looking up at the ceiling and let the others do the work.

No one else can be in the room with me for the treatment, just me and that gigantic, intimidating machine. I felt lonely, very lonely and sad. My tears came because of what was happening and I really needed someone to hold my hand and to feel what I felt.

The radiation lasted only two minutes and when it was finished, one of the nurses came in and gave me a hug. She told me this was the last step and that I had to stay strong, it's not easy but I came through it and now it's just 44 more to go, and she started laughing.

Dr. Jonathan Stella, is my radiologist, a very nice man, a very optimistic person. He gave me all the answers to my questions and he will see me once a week during my treatment, to make sure of my progress, and after I'm done I will see him every 6 months for follow up.

While I was waiting, I had my mother-in-law Norma, or my sister-in-law Sherri with me. Most of the time, they took turns in taking me to get my radiation. I am so grateful for them because I had somebody to talk to and distract me a little bit. I met a girl about my age, maybe a little older, who was to receive her final radiation, she started to tell me her case and it was much more complicated than mine. They had found cancer in her lymph nodes, and there was a possibility that the cancer would re-emerge in the same breast or the other one. She said her breast was burnt from the radiation and the pain was so intense that they had to postpone the treatment for a time. I honestly do not know how my body will react, but I will do everything possible to make it tolerable. I thought this couldn't be worse than chemo. I had so many questions for the doctor and he said the only thing I could do was to apply aloe vera lotion. I am prepared and with the help of God and my papa I'll come out of this, too.

After I had finished talking to the charming girl, I went to my car, sat down and thought my case could've been much worse and I must have faith that this treatment will be effective and that I won't have to go through all this again although I would if it meant I would live. What else can I do?

I maintained that attitude and conviction were my best weapon against cancer and I tried not to let the cancer dominate my life. Cancer is a menace and a threat in the life of a human beings and I will always carry it for the rest of my life. During this entire process, I have met so many people with different types of cancer and, for reasons I can understand now, people with cancer are stronger, less self-absorbed, interested and above all caring. Probably it is because these people, with or without knowing it, have come face-to-face with their own mortality, and the people I have met are remarkable with a great spirit and an enormous desire to live. Fortunately, I am one of them.

Fifteen days had passed, and I've noticed that my breast has turned darker, almost bronze. I feel some burning sensation, not bad, but somewhat uncomfortable. I can't wear a bra and anything touching my skin bothers me. Also the pain gets more intense daily.

After 23 three days of treatment, the pain was very intense, my breast is totally dark and the burning is now visible. At times, I would ask myself which was worse, chemo or radiation. With the chemo, the symptoms would go away after the fourth or fifth day but with the radiation, the pain had been continuous. It was like having a headache that you can't get rid of. I used aloe vera and all sorts of lotions to ease the pain sometimes just for a few minutes. I've cried so much and the only thing that kept me on my feet and moving forward was knowing that it was almost over. The fatigue was indescribable. The doctor had warned me, but I never imagined that it would be as strong as it was. I felt like an ancient person. Cleaning my house used to take about an hour and a half and now it takes me about four hours and then I'm completely exhausted.

My daughter would come home from school and wanted to go to the park, to play or just go for a walk, I went with her when I could, but the fatigue was so intense that I had to sit down with her and explain my situation. At that time, I didn't have my mom with me, and my husband would come home on the weekends, so I was completely alone and unable to do things with her during the week. I asked her to be patient, that it was almost over and of course she understood. It was difficult because for forty five days traveling for my treatments my life centered around my routine for radiation treatments, the same faces, the same patients, the same sadness and loneliness. I couldn't wait for my last day.

Finally, the long awaited day arrived. I came with gifts and thanked everyone. I got on the table, but this time, with a big smile on my face, I received my final treatment and, at last, with tears in my eyes I got up and hugged all the technicians and told them "my nightmare is over for now." I remember that I went to the dressing room, and I took a last look of all the drawers, I prayed for all the names that each drawer had and finally, took my name off my drawer. The nurses gave me a diploma for having finished my treatment satisfactorily.

This is a good way to end my story, and not every story has a happy ending. I am closing this chapter of my life, saying only that for now, this battle is won. I don't know what tomorrow will bring, my fears and memories will always be remembered, but that doesn't matter because:

Whatever happened yesterday will help me live a fuller life today, because tomorrow, tomorrow is not here yet.

Congratulations, you are an official graduate of
San Luis Radiation, Oncology.

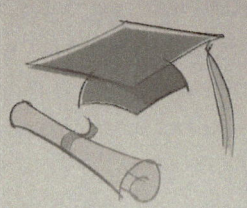

Presented to Dalia Burton
On this 15 *day of* September, *2006*
Dr. Stella, Dr. Chen and Staff.

One of the best day of my life

ABOUT THE AUTHOR

Dalia Burton, that's my name. I am just a simple and ordinary person who wants to help you understand how important it is to learn to know your body and all it's changes. That is how I discovered BREAST CANCER.

In this book, I wish to describe all of my experiences, hopes, dreams, loneliness and feelings in a simple manner, from the bottom of my heart. This is who I am, an ordinary woman who always likes to express how I feel without hidden feelings.

I am a woman with dreams and hopes who understands just how hard and fragile life is. I, at the age of 36, came to know that no matter how difficult life can be, as hard and hurtful as it may be, we must always bring out the positive side.

I am a woman who thought I had had difficult situations, who in some moment thought I had an insurmountable problem. I always saw those who were near as happy and content without any worries.

At times, we think that life is just getting up in the morning and going through our daily rituals. We never think how truly wonderful life is and know how to live, to enjoy the sunshine, the wind, the sea or simply sit in a comfortable chair or lie in bed and read a good book. Truly to know how to enjoy life is to enjoy it in the way we feel good and make us happy.

If we look around us, what do we see? Do we see insignificant things? We do hear our friends' stories, but are we listening? Sometimes we don't hear the song of a bird or the sound of a crystal clear river. We don't just sit and admire all the beauty that God has given us to enjoy.

It is in these little things that are, in fact, our whole world, where we live and grow. At times, our routine intoxicates us and when we have a problem or we come across a difficult situation unexpectedly, that is when we become aware that life is marvelous. There are things so much more important than triviality, anger, spite, things that surround us, and apathy. Yes, that's how it is, having tough times teaches us to be more human and to value life as it is, simple and wonderful.

We, as human beings, complicate life. If, as they say, the only life we've got, why don't we make everything that happens to us an experience? Make the best of it because that's how it is! This is how I learned to live and fight for those I love: without limits and being happy in spite of TOUGH TIMES.

978-0-595-49680-8
0-595-49680-6